# *IMPROVE YOUR SOCIAL SKILLS*

Stop Anxiety and Build Self-Esteem, Improve Your Social Life, Improve Relationship, Improve Self-Awareness. Make Friends and Talk to Anyone With High Level Conversation.

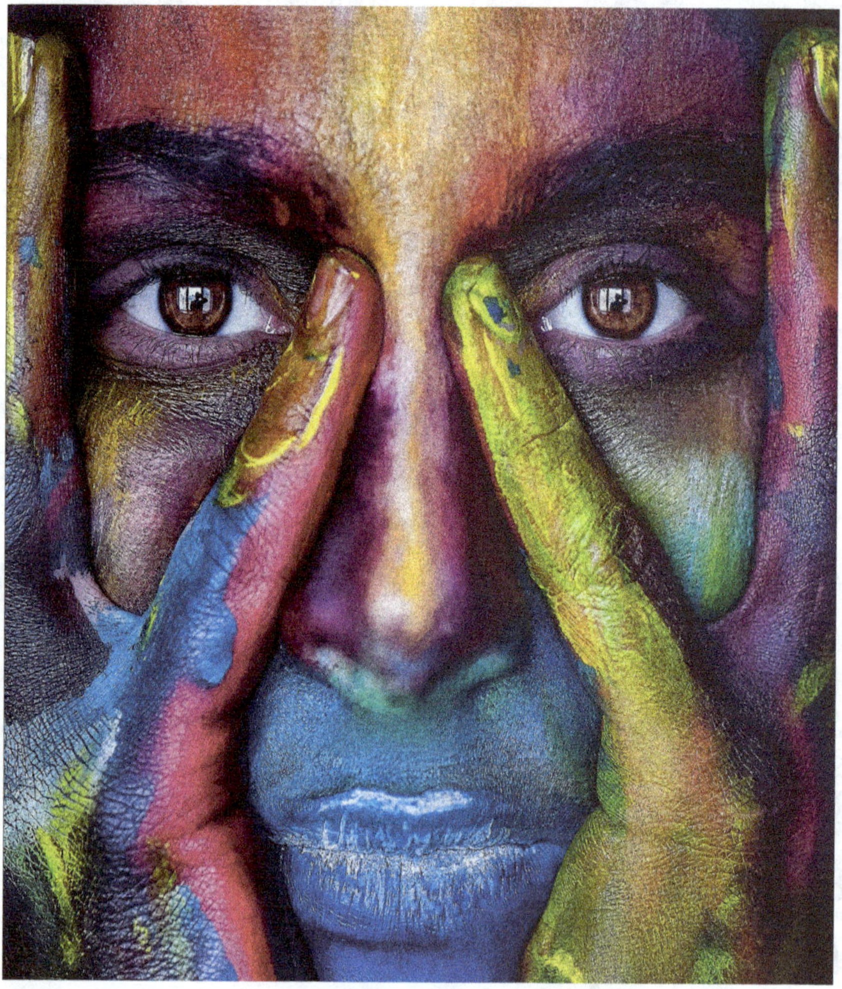

# Table of Contents

The information in the following pages is broadly considered a truthful and accurate account of facts and as such, any inattention, use, or misuse of the information in question by the reader will render any resulting actions solely under their purview. There are no scenarios in which the publisher or the original author of this work can be in any fashion deemed liable for any hardship or damages that may befall them after undertaking information described herein.

Additionally, the information in the following pages is intended only for informational purposes and should thus be thought of as universal. As befitting its nature, it is presented without assurance regarding its prolonged validity or interim quality. Trademarks that are mentioned are done without written consent and can in no way be considered an endorsement from the trademark holder.

# Introduction

Congratulations on purchasing "***Improve Your Social Skills,"*** and thank you for doing so. It is a social world, and downloading this book is a significant step towards improving your social skills. The first step is usually the easiest. All of the information contained herein is important for you to take to heart. These are not all concepts that you can immediately put into action. However, you can preserve this useful information for use at a later date. Of course, you will find it to be quite educational and worth putting into action in the future.

That being said, the chapters contained in this book will highlight and discuss some steps that are necessary to help you integrate seamlessly into society. This means you will start by learning how to think critically in a social way, and how you can act like a social person by changing your mindset from being antisocial, to an utterly social person. At the same time, you will learn the best way you can put your good manners into action to blend in well with others. Keep in mind that you will have to start gradually while getting integrated into the social circle, as well as adapting to the new environment, among other things.

There are volumes upon volumes of books on how to improve your social skills but thank you once more for selecting this one. Please enjoy!

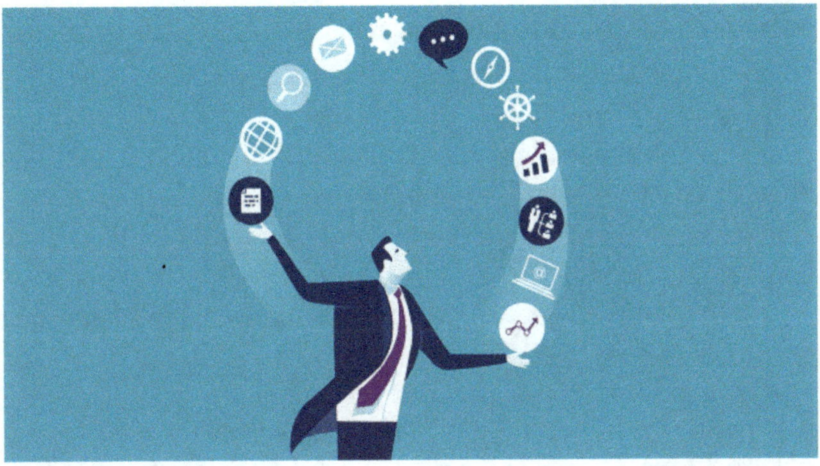

# Chapter 1: Think Socially and Act Like a Social Person

Social skills are more or less the same as any other skill you can learn in your life. This means that if you invest a little of your time and effort in studying and practicing such skills, you will get better as you gain experience. It doesn't matter where you come from, your environment or social status, which is essential in this regard. Anyone can acquire social skills, and it is never too late to do so. That is why your first step into learning social skills should be to think socially and act as a social person. And how do you even get started to achieve this feat?

## Think Socially

By nature, humans are social animals. This is evident from their behaviors, beliefs, and desires, which are always affected by the social preferences, their kind of interaction and social contexts that they live in. Human beings have evolved socially to become group-minded individuals who perceive everything in different perspectives. That is why they precisely understand what is in their minds or those around them, and act as though their brains are in sync with those of other people.

However, your ability and tendency to associate with like-minded people who collectively behave in a manner that seems desirable to you shows how you think socially. By associating with members of a group that think almost as you do can lead to affecting the decisions you make as well as your behavior, and this is crucial for your mental development.

Your social tendency as a human being is a clear indication that you are not purely selfish with sharing information and wealth maximization. Your ability to think socially means that you value fairness and reciprocity and that you are more than willing to cooperate in attaining shared goals. In the long run, you will develop a tendency to adhere to a common understanding and principles that will govern your behavior to benefit you or your group of like-minded individuals. After all, what you do will not only have a significant impact on you but also to those you usually interact with. And of course, your influence will change the behavior of everyone within your social circle by simply adopting your social thinking.

But there are consequences of thinking socially. A necessary result is, different groups comprising of like-minded people and even the societies across the board can adopt, and sadly stick to a particular collective pattern of behavior, such as segregation, corruption, supremacism and civil wars, that arguably benefit no one in particular.

On the other hand, the same tactics of social thinking can have a significant impact. Similar to social behavior, temporary interventions can lead to having a broad and everlasting positive outcome on a specific community through the shift in the pattern of social interactions. Also, social thinking can act as a lever for different types of development intervention that are likely going to harness the tendencies of individual groups to look for social status, maintain social identities and improve cooperation with other people under certain conditions. All these attributes come about when you or those within your group think socially, to develop your social skills.

There is an innate human desire for tendencies to be identified with certain groups and help one another in acquiring new social status and propensities to identify themselves with other people who are ready and willing to cooperate with them. As a human being, you can take full advantage of such desires and tendencies to advance your social skills by interacting with other people within your social network. This is because social networks play a crucial role in transmitting social influence to spur social change.

In addition to that, social networks are known to provide the right platforms where you will learn and adopt essential skills that can help you think socially. And one thing that will help you to realize such changes, is what is commonly referred to as social norms. Through social norms, you will be able to coordinate your behavior and adopt new principles that will guide you all along as you interact with others.

Just like a river flowing through a specific society, so is the human sociality. Its impact on the community is immeasurable, given that it influences everyone, shapes individuals, and helps them pursue a common goal in their daily undertakings. Now that you are part and parcel of that society, you can choose to follow the current or swim upstream but know that whichever decision you make it will have a positive or a negative impact in the end. For that reason, sociability will serve as a stepping stone to the new world of development interventions through which your social skills will play a very significant role.

One area that can help you tap into your potential in improving your social skills, lies in social networks. Although getting into search networks is an individual's decision, there is no better way of learning how to think socially than through a social network. As the world changes technologically, human beings are shifting from the traditional way of doing things to the modern way of life. This doesn't imply that these changes affect a handful of people but a multitude from different corners of the world.

The truth of the matter is that all of us are embedded in all kinds of networks that suit our needs. Of course, these are networks of our social relations that are tailored towards shaping our resources, beliefs, preferences, and choices we make in our daily lives. After some time, you will come to the full realization that any social network is a set of actors as well as relational ties, forming the very building blocks of your social experience. Why is the case?

The answer is simple and clear. Networks are essential platforms that provide different scopes with which individuals can reinforce existing human behavior among themselves. At the same time, these networks can help them in transmitting normative pressures and novel information that, at some point, will spark social change as a result of thinking socially. Apart from that, the ability of a social network to both shift and stabilize patterns of people's behavior indicate that they may play an essential role in their social settings in which formal institutions are not available.

Unfortunately, most people disregard social networks even though these are a foundational basis of any social order. And without a warrant, human beings can be rendered savages in all aspects of their behavior and how they relate to one another. So, socially thinking can overcome such negative human attributes and make the world a better place for everyone.

Socially thinking will help you blend in perfectly with people from different backgrounds and social status. Your sociability will enable you to break barriers and get influenced by new ideas coming from your social peers.

It will be a matter of time before you get to realize the importance of thinking collectively and sharing ideas that are constructive in the long run. On the other hand, selfishly acting will lock you out of many available opportunities.

It is evident that human behavior is diverse, and everyone chooses what is appropriate for them. But being antisocial or introvert can be a choice that will limit your social skills and deny you a golden opportunity to learn and share vital information with others. While some individuals come out to defend the idea of being anti-social, the ramifications of this vice outweigh the benefits in a social setup. It doesn't mean that the society is forcing you to adopt those ideas and norms that could go against your well-being, but it is only encouraging you to start thinking socially in order have a positive impact on your social skills.

It is true you that you may experience some negativities on your quest to acquiring the right social skills, but it doesn't mean you fall out along the way. When the going gets tough, the tough get going, and you need to overcome every barrier if you want to realize your potential. Nothing comes the easy way, but through persistence, you will understand how easy you will get to achieve your goals. Therefore, the first step to start improving your social skills lies in your ability to start thinking socially. In this way, your mind will be prepared adequately for what lies in the future, and by the time you reach the peak of all events, you will be in a better position to showcase your social ability.

But keep in mind that you cannot do it on your own unless you interact with individuals with whom you share common interests and are eager to learn from each other. Socially thinking means that you will soon start acting socially and return; your social skills will be on an entirely new level.

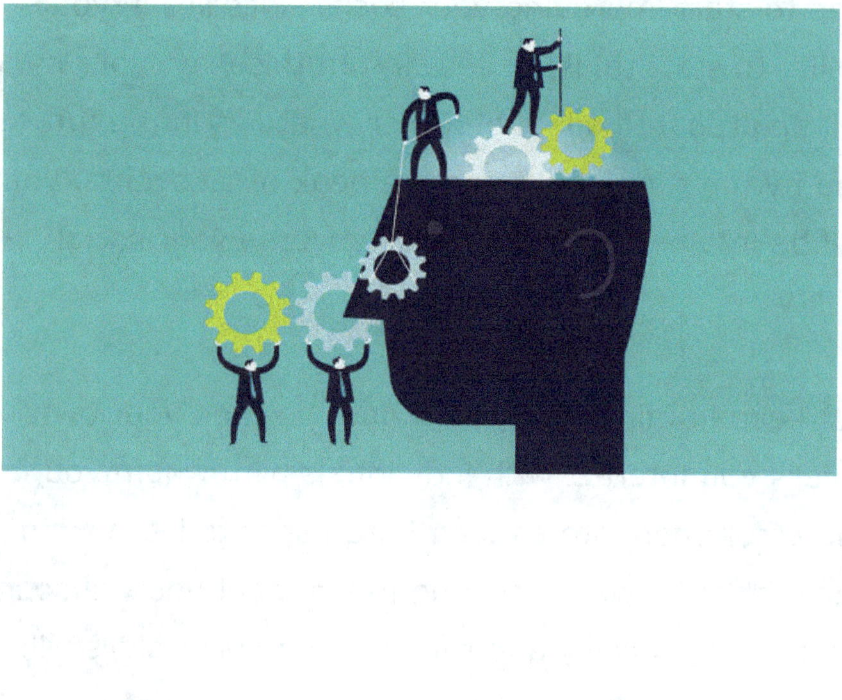

## Be comfortable with all strata of society

A socially skilled person can get along with people across all strata of society. Not necessarily every person, but every type of person. This is a useful skill, and it is also a significant benchmark. You could rely on commonality with a clone of yourself but must genuinely exercise your social skills when trying to relate to someone with whom you have little in common. If you cannot do that, then you may be skilled at relating to people with whom you are compatible with, but not be socially competent.

The commonality is a shortcut to rapport, and a good one to use if it is available. But sometimes the most interesting conversations and friendships happen between people with little commonality. After all, by definition, if you have less in common, there's more new territory to explore.

Building this skill requires travel outside of one's comfort zone, as well as grappling with hidden insecurity. On one end of the spectrum, it's possible to feel inferior to people you admire, as though you don't have any value to add to the relationship. On both ends, lack of commonality can be a hard barrier to cross, especially if it is apparent that you're from different backgrounds and the other person is intimidated by it.

Someone who is comfortable interacting and befriending people in all strata of society will feel comfortable in nearly every situation, confident in his ability to add to any interaction of which he's a part. He'll have more opportunities to share what he knows with others, as well as the ability to learn from experiences that he may never have personally.

## Be a net addition

Beyond just getting along with people in all strata of society, you want to generally be a net positive to any social situation in which you're placed. If someone was eating alone, and you were to join them, that should make their lunch better. If a few friends are having tea together, and you get invited, your presence should make everyone have a better time. And if you go to a large party or event, even though your impact will be proportionally smaller due to the size, those you interact with should be glad that you were at the party.

Most social circles are a series of concentric circles. There's the small inner nucleus of people who organize and get invited to everything, and without whom events wouldn't even happen. Then there's the next ring of people who are always welcome but would never displace a member of the nucleus. Outside of those two circles are people who usually get invited, but only if space permits. Or maybe they have specific personality quirks that make them incompatible with others in that circle, meaning the core group must choose who gets invited and who doesn't.

The nucleus is comprised of the people who are net additions, and who orchestrate events. The next circle is those who are also new additions. The circle further out are people who are "not negative." Sometimes they add, sometimes they're neutral. They're nice to have around, but not a, sure enough, the thing to make sure they come to every event. Beyond those rings are people who are sometimes or always net negatives.

By ensuring that you're always a net addition, even if you're not a huge one, you will dramatically increase the number of events to which you are invited. Besides being fun and valuable, these invitations will provide you with events at which you can practice your social skills, creating a virtuous.

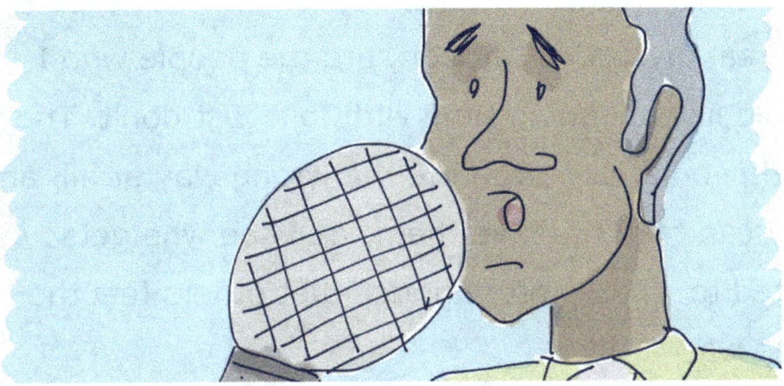

## Being dynamic

I probably shouldn't say this, as it will make just about everyone feel awkward around me, but I'm continually analyzing people's social skills. When I really like being around someone, I think a lot about why that so. There are some people whom I can spend weeks with and still be excited about their company. How do they do that?

The real mysteries, though, are the people who I should like spending time with, but just don't. They're good people, don't rub me the wrong way at all, and yet I can take or leave them; as I see who gets invited to what, I often notice that others feel the same way.
What do these people have in common? What can they do to shift the perception others have of them and be in a better position to share their positive aspects?

The best definition, loose as it is, is that these people lack the quality of being dynamic. They're predictable, reserved, and seem to endeavor to minimize their impact on others.

In my definition, I mean a particular type of being predictable. It's good to be predictably timely, cheerful, and any other number of positive attributes. But there's something really magnetic about someone who brings something different to the interaction every time. You don't know what they'll say. Maybe they'll have a fascinating question they're mulling over, perhaps a great new story, or maybe some exciting new place they've found. Their positive contribution to social interaction is unpredictable.

People who are reserved and minimize their impact succeed in leaving everyone unoffended, but people go to social gatherings for a reason, and that reason is not to be unoffended or remain un-impacted.

## Act Like a Social Person

You don't need some form of magic or a Ph.D. in rocket science to act as a social person. It all starts with you before getting influenced by other like-minded people. In this regard, your ability to think socially should motivate you to act like a social person if at all, you are ready to hone your social skills. And if you do it right soon or later, you will be on everyone's minds, and your sociability will pave the way to a world of opportunities.

You may get despaired or face some negativity from pessimists, but your courage and resilience will pay off ten-fold. You can start from a simple conversation with strangers to several chats to those who try to talk you all the way taking part in team-work activities among others. All these actions are meant to make you seem like a social person, and within no time, you will be one. So, let's find a way out to make your life quite enjoyable through acting as a social person.

## Initiate a constructive conversation with a stranger(s)

Taking the initiative to strike up a conversation requires enough courage and some wisdom because you are not sure of the response from the other party. But whatever the outcome, you should be fully prepared no matter what. However, your approach will lay a firm foundation for your conversation. A good strategy will lead to a meaningful discussion, but an immature one might culminate into an unpleasant situation that will leave you despaired or embarrassed all along. So, where do you start?

Greetings are known to break all barriers among different people and society's world over. Greetings are a sign of peace, friendliness, politeness, and good manners. Walk straight to your target audience and say "hello, nice meeting you and I are so and so…"

Even though the person you are trying to have a conversation with doesn't show signs of being interested in the first place, greetings will ultimately change that. If you are lucky enough, your discussion will mark the beginning of a very long relationship and a social network.

By the time you finish with greetings, you should know what comes next if at all, your intention is to initiate and maintain that particular conversation. Of course, you will introduce yourself formally, and by doing so, the tension between you and your immediate target will gradually start going down. This is the right time to break the ice and introduce the topic of your discussion.

It may sound easier said than done, but if you are well versed with what is happening around you, you will not fail to find a topic that both of you will enjoy discussing. You can think of sports, climate change, current affairs, or even politics if only you share a common approach on that.

Make your conversation an interesting one and let your new partner keep enjoying everything you say to stay relevant while gradually gaining more and more confidence. With time your friendly approach and ability to sustain a conversation will motivate you into talking to different people regardless of their social status, beliefs, age differences, culture, and background. A good discussion will create an everlasting impression to those you closely interact with, and in the end, you will suddenly come to realize that your social skills are paying off day by day and from person to person.

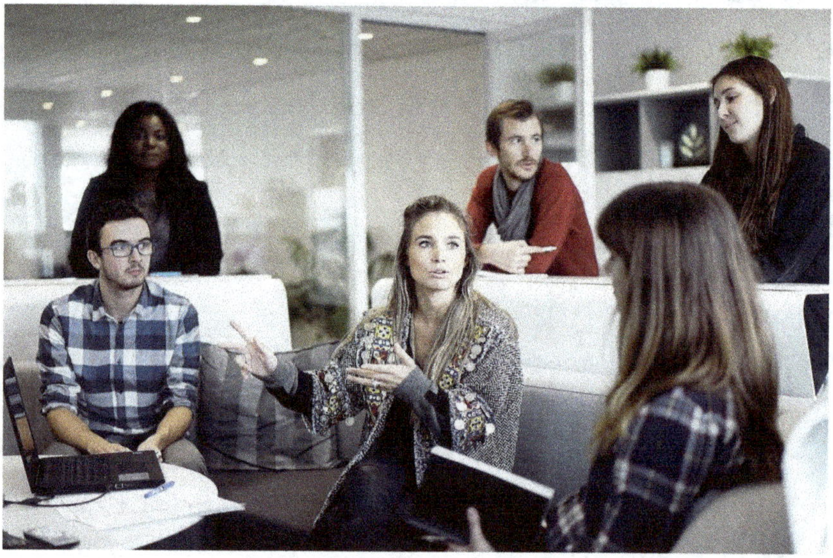

## Chat back to those who try to talk to you

Perhaps at one point, you might have tried talking to individuals you've just run into and they coldly respond to by their one-word response. For sure this sounds rude and paints you as someone out there to intrude others. Such unfortunate encounters are enough to discourage you, especially when it is your first time to try to engage someone in a conversation.

If other people around are trying to initiate a chat with you, it is polite of you to make an effort by giving them positive and meaningful responses in return. It won't cost you a thing, but you will stand to gain even more through that simple gesture. Besides, your social skills will improve significantly by learning how to handle different people in different situations verbally. Being selfish and self-centered will not help you in any way, and you will stand to lose a lot of good chances or opportunities if you have that terrible habit of snubbing other people.

## Take part in various group activities

There are numerous activities taking place around, and you can take a while from your busy schedule to participate in them. This is one area that you can sharpen your social skills through close interaction with people from different places and diverse backgrounds. Being part of an active group means that you and other members will spend much of your time discussing, issuing instructions, or giving suggestions where necessary. Doing so will help you in learning effective ways to communicate with your peers.

On the other hand, you may invite your friends, neighbors, family members, and even strangers to be part of your forthcoming event. It could be your birthday party, your wedding or even your fundraising event. At the height of your event, you will have that opportunity to express yourself, and there's no better way of doing so if not that your communication and social skills are top notches. It doesn't mean that you have to be a good speaker or crown mobilizer, but you can gradually learn as time goes by.

## Try to look like an outgoing person

Who doesn't like associating with celebrities? Of course, everyone wishes to be in the shoes of their favorite celebrities for one reason or the other. This is not to imply that you have to break your back, trying vehemently to look and behave like someone famous. What it means is that you need to look and act in a manner that will portray you as someone outgoing. And the best way to do so is through your social skills.

Being an outgoing person will give you enough confidence to face different people without fear of being intimidated or ridiculed, given that nearly all your friendly status will place you in a position almost similar to that of a celebrity. Now that you will be accorded such status, it will be upon you to take advantage of your near-celebrity status to improve your social skills. It may not be easy for you to attain such status overnight, but through self-determination and hard work, nothing will stand your way.

## Join other people where they are

They could be your workmates, family members or your fellow students you want to establish a close link with them. Ensure that you join them wherever they go and in what they are doing. If it is a lunch-hour or an evening stroll, you should always consider being part of that group so you may learn how to socialize with different people.

For instance, if you happen to be at a party, and almost everyone is talking at the front porch, compose yourself and join them to take part in what they might be discussing. Share your views on the topic of discussion and be ready to listen to others. Keeping to yourself will not do you any kind rather than denying you the chance to practice your social skills.

Even though being an introvert is not harmful in any way, it might look awkward to keep to yourself at a social gathering when everyone is jovial and to share one or two jokes. You will look out of place and consequently, get bored all along. Therefore, find the best way to approach other people and use that opportunity to improve your social skills.

## Spend some time with people

It is always important to spend some time with people as you learn their way of life and how they carry on with their activities. These could be your friends, neighbors or even workmates. Give them your quality time, and they will appreciate your effort in doing so.

Giving people much of your time should not be taken as a waste of your precious moment because every person you come across will influence you either positively or negatively. Whichever the case, it is upon you to make up your mind on what you are being impacted on.

As you spend more time with people, you will likely come across someone who will help you in changing the way you approach and socialize with others. Also, it will help you to learn better ways of handling different types of people given that every society has its uniqueness, so are its people. If your social skills are improving, it merely means that you are on the right track.

Thinking socially and acting as a social person is one step into the realms of a social world. Since no man is an island, it means that we need each other to survive, to share our happiness, triumph, sadness, story and even our achievements. There is no better way human beings can express themselves if not through socializing; hence the need to improve on our social skills. Therefore, start by thinking socially and acting like a social person and the world around you will be a better place to express yourself freely.

# I Have My Period

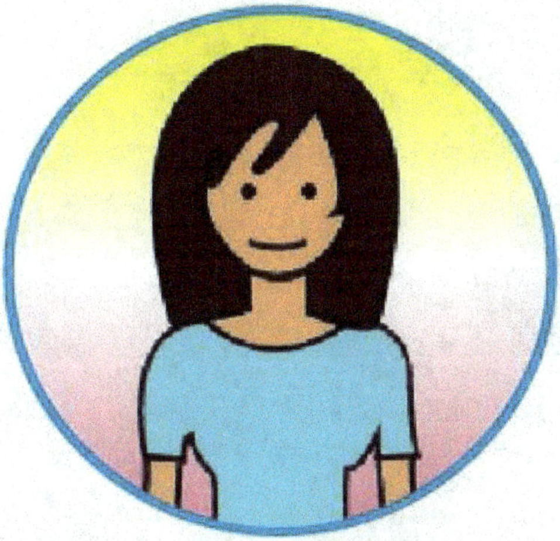

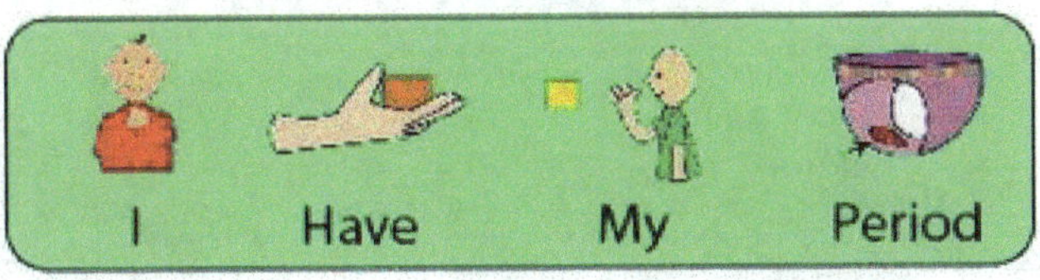

# Chapter 2: Learn and Apply Good Manners to Improve Your Social Skills

"Manners maketh man" is a famous quote from the movie, *'Kingsman: The Secret Service,"* and it merely means that their manners judge human beings. Without good manners, then the rest of humanity is savagery. Every society, individuals, and different institutions across the world will treat you according to your behaviors, let alone your physical appearance. Learning and applying good manners should be the first thing to do if you want to have a positive impact on your social skills.

The importance of having outstanding social skills cannot be overlooked right in the earliest years of childhood to a complete adult. Solid social skills play a very crucial role in shaping an individual as well as helping with personal relationships and career advancement.

There are many ways you can improve your social skills, and one of them is through learning and adopting good manners that will make you be accepted in society. From the basics of good manners to group activities, all the way to help bolster skills. If need be, you may seek outside assistance from professionals who will help establish a firm foundation for what is coming ahead of you.

## Explain Your Personal Space

One of the basics that you will need when learning good manners is to explain your own space. This is essential in helping you grasp the concept that those you will interact with, in the near future, have their space bubble, and they deserve respect from you.

To understand this concept fully, you will need to keep at the back of your mind that personal space varies from one individual to the next and from one culture to another. It will be upon you to take your time to understand those people who are closer to you. They could be your relatives, friends, school mates, parents, and your siblings.

For example, one group of individuals may be more comfortable with the idea of hugging and touching while the rest are used to just shaking hands and a simple peck on their cheeks or hands. This is because any given society comprises of different people and different cultures; thus the need to learn how you can approach everyone. In other words, some people may have varied preferences for personal space.

Still, on the personal space, you will need to go an extra mile to study everyone's body language keenly. Though it may sound like a complicated thing to learn, a body language is universal, and with the right knowledge about it, you can always interpret it from one person to the other.

The first signs you will have to look out for in a person you are trying to interact with will tell you if that particular person is interested or not. For instance, you may have come across a group of people or just an individual who portrays a sign of tensing up or crossing their arms and eventually backing away. This is a clear sign that you are infringing on their personal space, and they are uncomfortable about it. So, if you had prior knowledge of body language, you would not try to invade their space in the first place.

Likewise, you are also entitled to your personal space. And once you are pretty sure of this fact, you will not let anyone get into your space without your permission. Don't just let anyone hug you without your consent in the same way you wouldn't embrace other people without consenting to that idea. Just know that you have full authority over your own body in the same way as other people.

## Understand the Necessary Skills to Have a Good Conversation

If you have basic conversational skills, know that you are on the right path to social development. But for someone trying to learn good manners and applying them in a standard setup, this can be a daunting task. To begin with, you may not have any idea of where to start, and you will be likely to be prone to interrupting others in the middle of their conversation. On one side, you might be lacking the right skills to initiate a conversation between you and a stranger or those within your social circle.

However, you should not be worried anymore if your social skills are way below your expectations. Everything has a beginning, and from here, you will have basic ideas on how you can have good manners that will help you sharpen your social skills.

Almost all interactive moments start from somewhere, leading to something more meaningful and long-lasting. That is why you will begin by learning how to enter a conversation without interrupting others or appearing like an unwanted guest.

The first thing that you will need to do is to start with basic greetings. Greetings are known to be the first show of respect when you are about to engage a stranger in a conversation. Addresses break that barrier that generally exists between two groups of strangers and creates the first impression that other people will use to gauge your social manners.

A simple 'hi' or "How are you" can change the whole game, and you could be on your way to establishing a long lasting relationship with people you always perceive to be strangers. Or you can think of using non-verbal cues if you are not sure of the language to use when initiating that very first move in a conversation. You can start by nodding, waving, smiling and handshaking. Well, a handshake has been known to be the most effective form of nonverbal greeting, and it serves the purpose of easing the tension between you and the next person.

Listening and waiting for the other person to speak is a vital skill that you will need to hold a meaningful conversation. Looking at someone without interrupting their conversation is a show of respect and being interested in what is being discussed. But interjecting when someone is speaking can make you look disrespectful, especially when having a conversation with a stranger for the first time.

Learning to be assertive while having a conversation with someone is one of the best skills that can improve your sociability. To be assertive does not imply that you are aggressive, but it means you are making an inquiry of what you want your subject to respond directly and honestly. When you communicate assertively, you should not use insults, threats or excuses to drive your point home. Stick to your ethical principles and use a polite language with a friendly tone throughout your conversation.

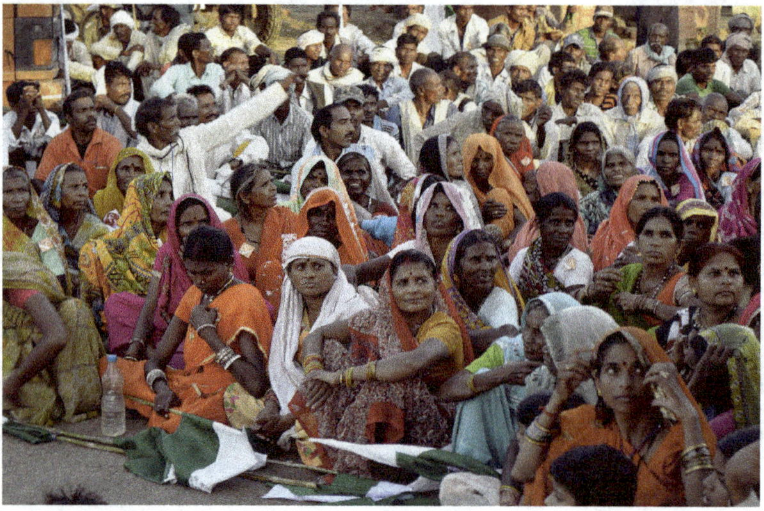

## Acquire Basic Manners

By now, you are old enough to understand good manners in general. However, you need to learn some basic behaviors that you can use to enhance your social skills. Using common phrases like thank you, please, excuse me, and all other forms of common courtesy can influence the way you interact with other people. Make these phrases to be part and parcel of your conversation as a way to convey good manners to those around you. Once this becomes a habit in your speech or communication, you will eventually come to realize how polished your social skills have grown. As the saying goes, "practice makes perfect," and you may capitalize on that if you want to stay in the game.

Basic manners don't just limit you to use polite words or phrases but go as far as employing the use of other equally critical social skills. One of the best skills that show how honest or interested you are in a conversation is the use of eye contact. It is understandable that there are shy people, and you could be one of them but maintaining eye contact with your subject will install a sense of confidence in you while making your conversation worthwhile.

Learning and adopting good manners goes beyond holding a constructive conversation with someone. Remember, table manners are also part of your social skills and one of the best etiquettes at meal time. Good behavior will make you stand out among the rest, and everyone will want to associate with you all the time. Before taking meals, especially when you are a guest, it is prudent that you start with observing your hygiene. Wash your hands thoroughly before meals, don't speak in between mouthfuls, place your napkin on your lap, use polite language and gestures while at the table with other guests and always remember to clear your dishes from the dining table.

Patience is not common among individuals, but it is also part of basic manners. Being impatience with others will not go down well, and you may end up being snubbed, or your presence assumed completely. Of course, you will not take it in kind if others treat you in a manner that will lower self-esteem. To avoid such awkward moments in a social gathering, practice patience and tolerance and learn what others expect from you so that your interaction with them will run smoothly. In addition to that, showing some elements of indulgence to your friends and family members will mean that you care and consider others in what you do. This is because human beings are a unique lot, and their reactions to different social situations might not be the same.

---

## Eliminating Annoyance

Before you begin working on how to bring a lot to the table, as a friend and a member of a friend group, it is essential to work on eliminating behaviors which annoy. None of us will ultimately succeed in removing all our annoying behaviors, but there's a certain threshold that must be crossed for people with other good options to choose you as a friend.

This is a harsh thing to say, but that doesn't make it untrue. Some of those you will most want to become friends with will already have a ton of good friends who are all competing for their time. If you have annoying habits, there's no guarantee that a new friend or acquaintance will be able to see past those habits and discover the great things about you.

A classic example is talking too much about things that the other person isn't interested in. There are guidelines to follow on how much of the conversation should be you listening versus you speaking, but in general volume alone won't make or break an interaction. After all, even if you prefer being the one to talk, if I'm revealing interesting discoveries about subjects that matter to you, you're unlikely to want me to stop.

But if I'm talking about my ambitions as a marathoner, and you have no interest in running, your capacity to enjoyably listen to me is limited.
Another common annoying habit is making bad jokes. No one thinks that they make bad jokes, but everyone knows some people that do, so there's an apparent disconnect. Some people consistently make bad jokes and don't realize it. You might be one of these people.

Both of these are undesirable traits, not because you're malicious or because they imply something wrong about you, but because they create an unnecessary imposition on the other person, and require him to either deceive you or be rude.

If you talk too much to me about subjects in which I have no interest, I must be polite, listen, and feign interest. The only alternative is for me to be rude, either by changing the subject as abruptly as I can manage or by telling you I'm not interested. Some people are so oblivious about overtaking that they won't pick up on any subtle cues make you aware that your jokes aren't funny. In either scenario, you've placed an awkward imposition upon me, making me less comfortable, less interested in the conversation, and more motivated to exit.

Identifying annoying habits is more difficult than eliminating them. Often awareness creates enough social pressure to at least dampen the annoying habit. If you have a friend or family member who is willing to be completely honest with you, you can ask them what annoying habits you have. Don't ask if you have any, assume that you do, and ask what they are. This saves your friend the awkward step of revealing to you that you have some.

Think about how often you'd be wrong when pointing out someone else's annoying habit. Probably rarely to never, so when someone gives you that sort of feedback, assume that they are correct.

You will have to find some annoying habits on your own, though. The biggest red flag is when you are consistently getting reactions that differ from those you expect. You make a joke, and the laughter is muted. You talk about something that interesting to you, but you see eyes wander and notice that your listeners don't ask any clarifying questions.

These are just two examples of many. Others include overuse of certain words, unnecessary hand gestures, not making eye contact, and not listening.

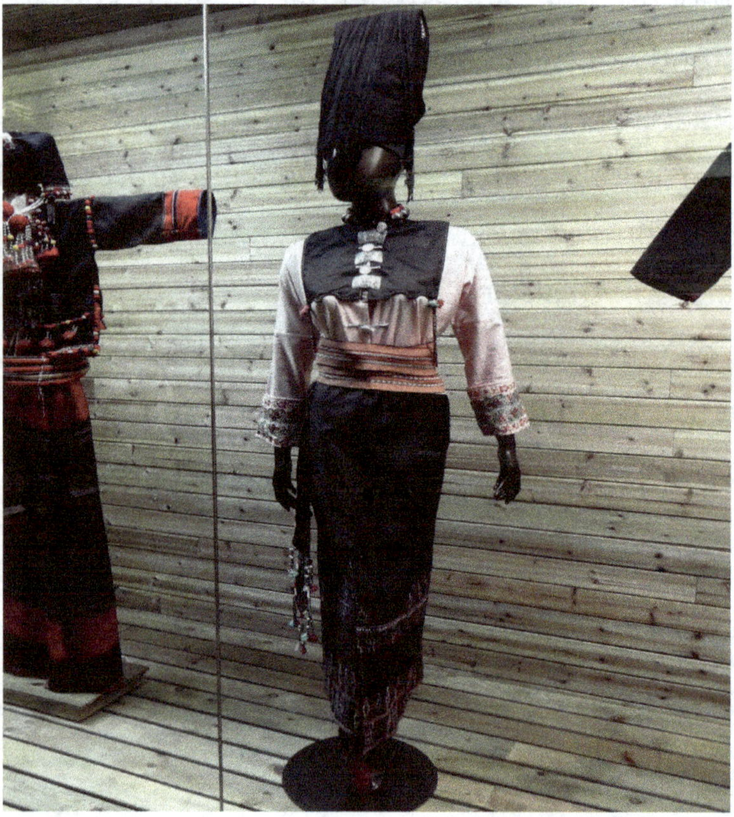

## Take Your Interest in Any Activity that Promotes Social Skills

A great way to help you model your social skills is by developing an interest in any action that is likely to encourage social behavior. There are hundreds of activities that you may engage in to improve your social skills. One of them is taking part in games where you will meet different people learn one or more things from each other. Games or sports bring people together, and this is one area to achieve scores of people with whom you probably share a common interest. If you are not a social person, taking part in such activities will change your social life as well as your perspective about other people.

Apart from that, you can also look further and reach out to those games that are explicitly designed to encourage conversations regarding social skills. Through such games, you will sharpen your conversational skills as well as your analytical thinking. This is one area you should consider given that it will expose you to various activities that will compel you y to engage other people in a one-on-one conversation. In the end, your shyness and introvert behavior will drastically change to something more meaningful.

According to the research, critical social skills such as leadership and empathy are usually learned during participation in various games. This means that when you show an interest in a specific game, you will need to find a way to be part of it. These games will have a positive impact on your overall social skills, besides engaging in physical activities to keep you healthy, both physically and mentally. The same research suggests that those people who start participating in team sports are less likely to abuse harmful substances and that they stand a good chance of having better self-esteem. However, you should not limit all your thoughts to sports even if your interest is not there. There are hundreds upon hundreds of other activities that can help you realize your potential in various fields of endeavor with social skills being one of them.

Other activities that can transform you into a social person include religious gatherings, picnics, going out to a club or an event with friends, and taking part in voluntary services within your residential areas. All these activities will make you meet many people, and you will not miss out on establishing some friendship with a couple of them in the course of your interaction.

## Seek External Support, if Necessary

It is not a bad idea to go looking for outside assistance in a bid to improve your social skills. This is necessary because at one point in your life, you will realize that you need to establish a close relationship with others to experience mutual benefit. As stated earlier, human beings are different, and their way of developing varies from one individual to the other. Some people have no problem with acquiring necessary social skills while others find it quite taxing to socialize with those around them. Since we are all in a typical setup, it will be awkward to lack basic skills that will enable you to mingle with others.

But there comes a time when your social development is way below your age mates, and however much you try to acquire those skills, nothing comes your way. Maybe your inability to develop socially is a sign that there is something different about you hence the need for some intervention. It could be some conditions such as autism or genetic disabilities that are hindering you from becoming a complete person in a given social setup.

It doesn't mean that you sit back and accept your fate as it is, but you can find an immediate remedy to help you lead a normal life. Seek advice and help from a psychiatrist if you are finding it hard to get along with others or not being able to recognize pictures or figures of familiar objects and so on. All these could be signs of someone whose social development is slow, or it is happening at an uneven pace. Accessing the right help in time can save you the agony of being in perpetual isolation.

## Look for a Mentor

There are many ways you can nurture your manners with the aim of improving your social skills. Since human beings learn from each other, it will be a sound idea to look for someone who will help you in nurturing your manners towards attaining proper and well-polished social skills. Having a good mentor around you will significantly impact your social behavior by copying and applying what your mentors teach you. Most people feel appreciated whenever they get someone to hold their hand and guide them in the right direction. When coupled with a positive attitude, you will undoubtedly be surprised how fast you will start catching up with every step your mentor helps to undertake. But remember your will-power to learn, adapt, and apply good manners is the only factor that will determine your social behavior.

Another important thing about having a mentor beside you is that you will get some encouragement, and giving up along the way will not be an option for you. When reinforced with valuable teaching tools, you will not have to spend more time grasping one or two concepts that you will need to apply to change the course of your social behavior.

A good mentor means a lot when it comes to transforming someone from being anti-social or clueless about interacting with others to being an all-round extrovert who can fit in any society perfectly. With a seasoned mentor on good manners that can help you improve your social skills, you will be at a more significant advantage of learning admirable traits such as helpfulness, kindness, cooperation, politeness, patience, honesty, altruism, consideration, compassion, empathy, graciousness and gentleness. If you can attain a handful of such traits, there will be no society that you won't fit in unless it is a hostile one. All these traits are geared towards making you a complete person full of attributes that others will find desirable. When combined, all these traits will give you essential skills to participate comfortably in any activity within your community and beyond.

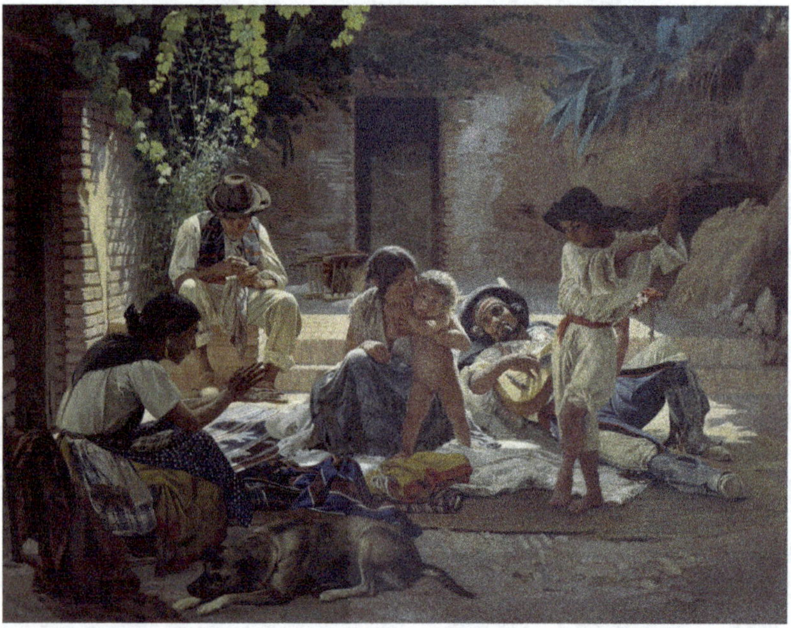

## Master the Art of Social Dynamics

Mastering the art of social dynamics entails quite a lot of steps when learning how to behave when applying good manners. First of all, you will need to start by building the knowledge, the like and the trust factor with your colleagues, potential friends, clients and even your boss ( if you are in a work environment). The art of social dynamism should help you to conquer all available networks by applying a better strategy that will take you from one stage to the next. To achieve that feat, you will have to master your conversations to appear competent and intelligent during your interaction with like-minded individuals.

By mastering the art of social dynamics, you will be setting a good platform that will enable you to maneuver your way into different groups of people with ease. This is not possible unless you have acquired basic manners that you can apply in any situation to blend in well with others. In the real sense, social dynamics will keep you on the right track and ahead of the game when it comes to associating with all types of people.

In a nutshell, your good manners will always create the first impression of you whenever you meet and have a conversation with new people. Your physical appearance may play a role, but not as much as your manners and everyone will judge you based on that. Sadly we all live in a judgmental world, and everyone you will come into contact with will judge you according to your deeds. Of course, nothing brings forth our acts better if not through the way we behave. Our behavior is the sole determinant of who we are and how we are treated. There are countless ways that you can learn good social manners. All these include; explaining your personal space, acquiring basic manners, showing particular interest in those activities that promote social skills, seeking to help from a mentor to mastering the art of social dynamics. These are some of the best ways that you can learn how to carry yourself when interacting with others at any common setup. Therefore, learning and applying good manners should be one of the vital steps that you can take to improve your social skills.

# Chapter 3: Start off Gradually to Acquire Social Skills

Everything has a starting point, so does your quest to improve your social skills. The truth of the matter is that no one was born with all the necessary social skills. Since life is a learning process, most of those you perceive to be socially endowed started from somewhere and grew to master these vital skills at their different stages of development.

Being of a certain age does not imply that you cannot start gradually and become a pro in socializing. Just give yourself some hope knowing that it is never too late to achieve your dreams. What you need is self-determination, the will power and the right platform on which you will launch your campaign to transform from being an introvert to a social person. So, where do you even get started?

Naturally, those perceived to be social didn't just wake up and found their way at the top of the social pyramid. They started from somewhere building up their confidence and social skills gradually. However, there are various places you can frequent in your free time to learn one or two tricks that can help you become a complete social person. These places include clubs, bars, restaurants, parties, public functions, schools, colleges and even religious gatherings, among others. Different people choose places that suit them or make them feel comfortable when mingling with others. What is essential in this regard is determining what works well for you.

Some people think that we are evolutionarily hardwired to evade situations with many strangers for safety reasons. While this notion is correct, it doesn't mean that we cannot approach strangers to establish a long-standing relationship. You can only know how social you are by mingling with people you hardly know and striking a constructive conversation. That is what makes other people look naturally social as compared to others. And that leads us to look critically into what it entails to be a typically socially successful person. Perhaps you are one of those lucky few to be social, but you are not yet sure about yourself. If you are not, you will consider looking for a conducive environment where you will feel comfortable in any social situation. In the actual sense, such an environment will help you to recreate the social path that will eventually lead you to other new avenues.

It will not surprise you to realize that the person with whom you perceive to be outgoing started right from kindergarten. As the years went by, the person in question nurtured the right skills, both communication and interactive, to become naturally socially. You too can identify the right spot to pitch your tent and work from nothing to something as far as becoming a social person entails. All that you need to do is have courage, the will, and determination, and everything will work in your favor.

This can sound obvious to you when presented this way, but upon seeing socially successful people interacting with others might not look that simple and obvious. Of course, you will feel disillusioned and then decide to give up prematurely. But before you call it to quit, always remember that fortune favors the bold. Be courageous and face any obstacle that might come your way. Don't dwell on an unsubstantiated belief that some people are born to be more successful than others. Nature does not allow that unless there is some amount of hard work involved. Therefore, every time you see a socially successful person in action, try to imagine the amount of effort and time they invested in achieving their target. You too can be like them only if you gather your courage and face any challenges coming your way.

On the other hand, it is essential to have an idea of the process involved when building social skills as well as confidence. Just in the same way, those socially successful people worked so hard to attain their current status, so should you. If others can do it, you too have what it takes to do it even better.

Start gradually by discovering those social situations that you think are a little bit thrilling but are still worth the struggle. Sit back and draw a plan that will guide you to overcome those thrills in whatever social situation you find yourself in. For example, you are used to enjoying parties in a company of a good friend that you have full trust in. But in the absence of your friend, the situation gets different directly because you cannot compose yourself and face strangers or mingle with people you do not know. To emerge a socially endowed person, you might consider taking the bull by the horns and face the situation as it comes.

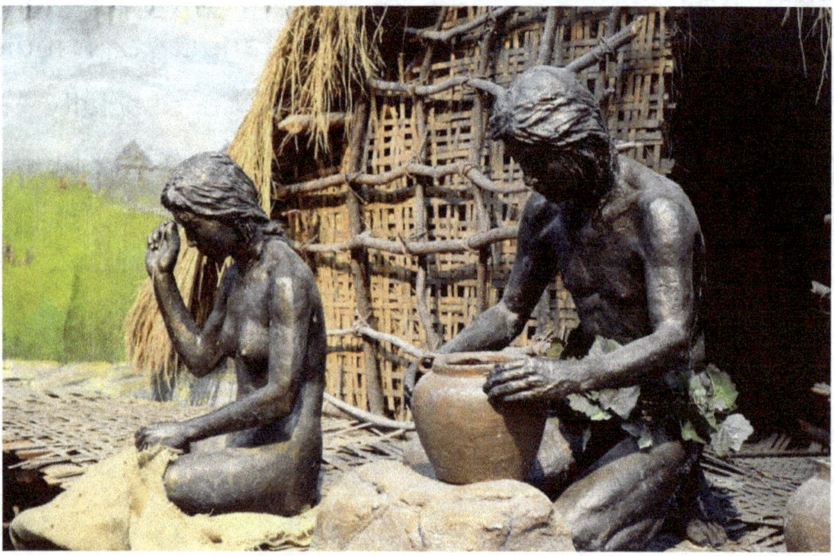

One beautiful evening you can choose to attend the party on your own in the absence of your closest friend and see how things will unfold for you. That will be the right moment to unleash your potential and overcome your fears. You never know the outcome, but with the right attitude and overcoming your concerns, you may find it quite easy to socialize with others without necessarily looking upon your friend to give you some courage. That is one way of starting to improve your social skills. Don't stop there and feel that you have finally achieved your dream. Just keep in your mind that there is more to come hence the need to be fully prepared.

Another perfect example is joining a meetup or a club for what you enjoy doing. Maybe it could be a meetup with your fellow entrepreneurs or athletes with a common interest in enhancing your talent. Take advantage of such meetings to further your social skills. Let others see you as an active person through your full participation in crucial matters affecting your organization or team and give suggestions where necessary.

In the actual sense, doing so will make profound differences between changing your current situation to become who you wish to be and forever remaining the same. As time passes by, these situations will gradually start feeling more natural, leading you to take entirely new steps. This doesn't mean that your task is already accomplished, but it instead gives you an excellent platform to advance your social skills.

## Levels of Communication

The cable that comes into your home for TV has only two wires running through it. The cable itself is a fundamental piece of technology that can be understood by anyone. But through this simple medium, hundreds of channels, as well as access to the entire internet, are transmitted. A lot is happening simultaneously.

This is very similar to how we communicate. Our words may seem very simple, but there are several different channels of communication being transmitted at the same time. To master social skills, you must be aware of these channels, be able to communicate effectively on them, and be able to understand what is being transmitted to you over them.

Four main channels are being communicated on at all times: content, Meta, emotion, and status.

Content is what we think of when we talk about communication superficially. If you tell me that you're going to the store, the content channel is merely telling me that you are going to travel to the store.

The meta-channel is the undercurrent of the conversation. It's the meaning behind the meaning--the implication. If we had been talking about how I wanted to eat brownies, and you're going to the store, the meta-channel communication is that you're going to get ingredients to make me brownies. Sometimes Meta can be read in isolation, but it usually requires context.

The emotion channel is more of a passive signal than an active circuit. Those of us who are not expert poker players are continuously leaking out our emotions as we speak. You could say, "I'm going to the store" in any number of tones and cadences. You could indicate that you were going to the store in resignation because I wouldn't stop hounding you about making me brownies. You could suggest that you loved me, and that's why you were going to get ingredients to make me brownies. You could also reveal that you were frustrated, nervous, excited, or any other number of emotions.

And last, the status channel is continually sending out clues about our relative status. If I were your boss and told you to go make brownies, you could say, "I'm going to the store" as an affirmation that you understood my command, and we're going to comply with it. You could also say it in a condescending tone that indicates that you're going to do it because I'm so far below you that I'm incapable of doing such an essential task myself.

I'm going to the store. Five essential words, chosen at random that could mean just about anything, even though the content doesn't change. If you weren't already awed at the power of communication, this might do it. It is incredible how much can be conveyed simultaneously.

A master of communication must be able to have two meaningful conversations (content and Meta) while maintaining two minor conversations (emotion and status). This is no exaggeration. If someone were to transcribe the Meta conversation between you and another person, it should be coherent. Same with the other two. If that conversation did not flow as smoothly as the content channel, you'd find that the conversation was frustrating to one or both of you, even if you couldn't identify why.

Each channel has its strengths and weaknesses, so when it's vital to convey something, you need to choose the right channel to focus on. I'll spare you a discussion on the content channel since you're able to understand it if you're able to read this book, but the other three channels deserve individual attention, especially since the most critical aspects of conversation happen in the channels hidden behind the content channel.

## Meta

The meta-channel may be the most important of the four. It's where real discussions happen. Sometimes you intentionally communicate incorrect information on the content channel, through sarcasm or joking, allowing your real message to come through on Meta.

The critical thing to understand about the meta-channel is that it's running all the time. People you speak with will always be wondering what you mean.

Let's say that you suggested that a group eat pizza. A couple of people agree to do so, and then another person says, "I guess I could do pizza." What he's communicating on the meta-channel is that he is willing to conform to group consensus and eat pizza, but that he'd rather eat somewhere else.

Now people answering after him can take that information into account when forming their responses. If the next person says, "Pizza sounds good," he's communicating a strong preference for pizza. He's ignoring the meta-message from the previous person. If he were less interested in pizza, the Meta communication from the previous person gave him the opportunity to begin shifting opinion. He could have said, "I could do pizza, or something else."

Once everyone answers, you have a good idea of how everyone in the group feels about it, but you still have options. If people hesitantly agreed and communicated on the meta-channel that they'd instead go somewhere else, you could have switched plans.

You might wonder what the point of this all is, especially if you're a very logical person. Indeed, it would be easier to communicate facts in the content channel and have no meta-channel.

The point of the meta-channel is that it allows for shades of gray not afforded by the content channel. If the content channel is a lecture, the meta-channel is a dance. It's pushing and pulling, circling and parrying. Imagine if someone said, "I'll eat at the pizza place, but I'd rather go somewhere else." That's what our first-person precisely communicated on Meta, but when it's in the content channel, it means something different. It's a much stronger disagreement and is the beginning of a disharmonious decision-making process.

Communicating on the meta-channel also allows people to save face. Let's say you met someone and liked them. They said that they want to see a Vermeer exhibit at a local museum. Their meta-channel is a bit unclear. Maybe they're inviting you, or perhaps they're not. You reply that you've also been wanting to see that same exhibit. Now you're communicating that you're not sure if it's an invitation, but that you'd like to go. If they aren't crazy about you, they can start talking about Vermeer, and thus communicate that they don't want to go with you. You can continue to have a civil conversation and not feel insulted.

If you instead focus on the content channel and say, "Hmm... I'm not sure if you're inviting me or not, but I'd like to go," you put them in a very awkward position. This is the exact type of conversation that should happen over the meta-channel so that neither person is made to feel bad.

Once you are tuned into the meta-channel, you might feel as though you are in the matrix. Even when people don't intend to communicate on the meta-channel, you can infer their sub-communications. You understand not just the "what" of people are saying, but also the way, and you gain the power to have two complete conversations at the same time.

The first step to communicating on the meta-channel is to continually ask yourself why people are saying the things they say. Why did he choose that exact phrasing? Why didn't she say something else instead? Why share that information now? Come up with some ideas in your head, and check them later when you have more information. By making predictions and verifying their accuracy then, you'll begin to calibrate your brain. When a prediction was off its mark, take the time to analyze and think about it.

Once you understand meta-communication, you want to start shaping yours. What we say can be interpreted in many different ways, so you have to craft what you speak for the specific person you're with whom you're talking. Try to create a simulator in your brain where, as you consider what to say, you predict how the listener will react, and what meaning they'll assign to it.

Sometimes when I read a non-fiction book, I decided that no matter what, I'm going to at least make one change as a result. I hope for a big breakthrough, but even a small tip can make a book worth reading. If you were to decide to do that with this book, I'd recommend having that change be focused on communicating more through the meta-channel.

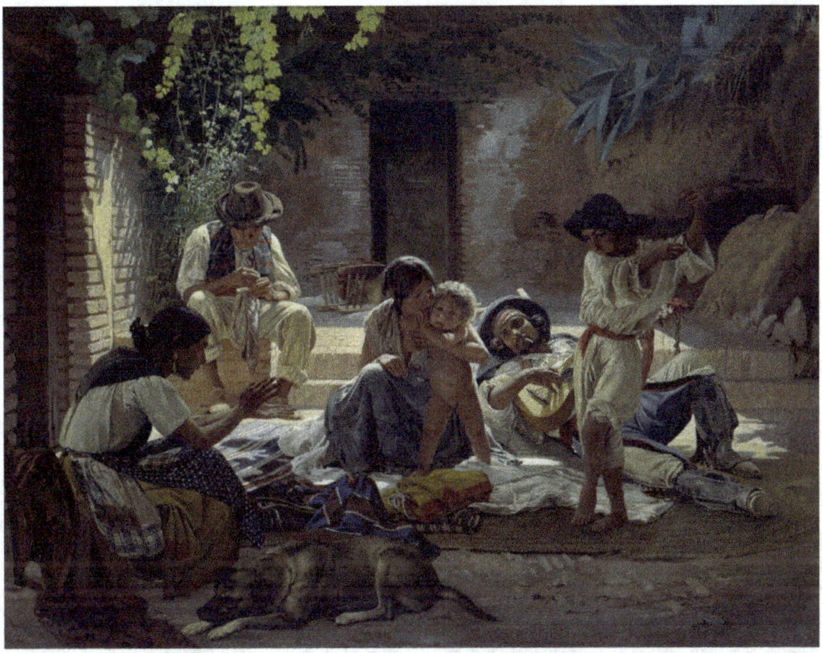

## Emotion

A lot of conversing is taking the other person on an emotional journey. You think about where they are emotional, as well as where they want to be, and you use the emotional channel to guide them there or keep them there if they're going to stay in the same place.

For example, let's say you meet someone at a concert. They're excited and having fun, which precisely is why they are at the show, so they want to maintain that state. If you initiate a severe talk about business, you are grossly miscommunicating on the emotional channel. Even if they enjoy business and being serious, it's so inappropriate in this context that they'll retreat from the conversation.

On the other hand, you could probably talk about business in an excited tone, and they'd engage with the conversation. The exact context would dictate whether it would work or not, but it's clear that it's a lot better than trying to be serious.

Consider someone who had a bad day and is frustrated. They probably want to shift to being happy and calm. You can slowly lead them in that direction by making the conversation increasingly positive. Maybe you'd start by matching their tone and asking them questions about the day, and then slowly bring some optimism to the discussion.
On the other hand, if someone were upset because they had a death in the family, though, they probably don't want to be happy. It just feels wrong. Maybe they want to feel understood and supported. You could communicate those things emotionally by listening, asking questions, and offering to do things to help.

Not every conversation is spiked with emotion, but there's usually some emotion there. If it's boredom, you've got to change that as soon as you can. If you're getting to know someone, maybe you'd want to emotionally communicate a little bit of mystery about yourself as well as excitement about getting to know them. Be aware of the emotional tone of the conversation and think about the directions you could move that emotion.

## Status

There is an invisible hierarchy in every group of people from two on up. If a decision had to be made, who would make it? If there were a crisis, to whom would people in the group turn to solve it? Who has to be more careful about what they say?

Humans are hierarchical creatures. We want to know where we stand, not for vanity, but to inform how we speak and act.

I could propose any combination of your friends, and you could probably sketch out a hierarchy. Maybe it would be flat, everyone being a peer, but more likely there would be a leader or two who get spoken to with just a tiny bit more deference and take more responsibility for the group. Whatever the hierarchy, everyone in the group would probably unconsciously agree to it and act and speak accordingly.

When you join another companion gathering, you need to comprehend the chain of importance. As a pariah, it's fundamental to keep up the concordance of the group, and not irritate it. If you know how the individuals identify with one another, that will be much simpler to do. Indeed, even one on one, status is essential. Understanding somebody's status is seeing how they see their place on the globe.

And, of course, you want to communicate your status. Some people will treat everyone with respect, but others only treat people with respect if they demand it. So your default outgoing communication on the status channel with someone new should usually be that you deserve respect and are worth getting to know.

A lot of statuses is communicated nonverbally with body language and eye contact. Direct eye contact conveys high status universally. Taking up a lot of space with your body also conveys high status.

Talking about how high status you are conveys low status. So does doing almost anything that is inappropriate in context. If you take up a lot of space where there's space to spare, you will appear to be high-status. If you take up a lot of space on a train where there are people who want to sit down, you look insecure and hard.

Vocal tone also communicates a lot about status. Someone who talks slightly louder than average and with clarity will appear to be more critical.

Instinctively reading status from the way people act and speak is consistent and accurate, which indicates that it's harsh to fake. If you feel like someone is high status, they probably are. If you think they're overreaching and are trying to convince you that they're high status, they probably are faking.
For this reason, it's dangerous to try to fake your status through body language and tonality. As you become more comfortable and confident, these aspects of communication will naturally change positively.

However, much of status is about what you will and won't accept from yourself and others. That can't be faked, but it can be changed. For example, many people will agree with higher status people as a blanket policy. Your boss says that he thinks the food at a restaurant is terrible, and you agree with him even though you think it's great. The "cool guy" at a party loves a song, and suddenly everyone likes it, too. This is a low-status behavior that invites disrespect.

Disagreeing with everything is even worse, but expressing your own opinion in a clear and appropriate way conveys that you can think for yourself, even in the presence of strong outside influence. You will be given respect for doing this.

Another primary changeable status indicator is whether you take responsibility or not. If you're at a restaurant and someone needs to speak to the waiter about moving some tables together, are you the one who does so? When a conversation is flagging, do you take the initiative and revive it? Ever-so-surprisingly, being a leader, indicates to others that you are, in fact, a leader.

Be aware of what others are communicating on the status channel, and avoid mannerisms or habits that accidentally convey lower status. In general, you should be communicating that you are a peer to people with whom you want to become friends. If you feel like someone is making an effort to appear higher status than you, it's sometimes worth taking action like speaking louder and taking up more space to place yourself a hair above them, only because they've indicated that status is important to them and that they respond to a higher status.

---

## Shifting Attentional Focus

A group of scientists was able to establish that when some test subjects were instructed to lay their focus on the people they were having a conversation with rather than themselves, it was found that they felt 67 percent more confident than before. These findings, when adopted, can help someone to start building their social skills step by step. Meaning that when you find yourself in any social situation, you should always try to focus on the person you are talking to, rather than yourself.

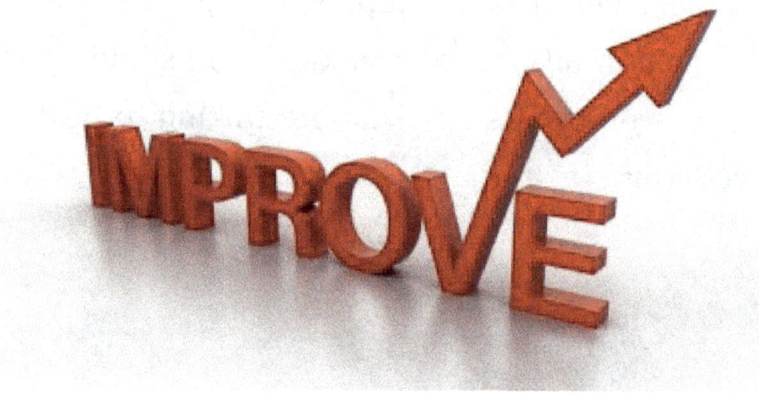
IMPROVE

If you keep on repeating the same action, you will come to notice how your mind shifts and starts focusing inwards thoughts such as "I'm now getting nervous" or "someone is thinking that I am awkward" and so on. While all these are common occurrences for someone who is trying to master social skills, it doesn't mean that you let those thoughts hinder your progress to becoming an all-around person. When it happens that way, you can save the situation by simply forcing yourself to start asking yourself questions regarding those around you instead. Questions such as "What are they working with?" "If she's an artist as she claims, what kind of art is that?" "How is he going to spend his free time?" and many more can considerably have a positive impact when it comes to shifting your attentional focus.

When your head is filled up with questions about others, it will take you a while to get used to those questions, but with enough practice, everything will happen automatically. Your brain will become less self-aware, making you more self-confident in the course of learning how to become socially endowed. Not only that. Also, you will have numerous questions lingering in your mind about how you can hold a constructive conversation with other people without necessarily losing your focus on attention.

Alternatively, you may move your conversation forward by asking those around you the questions that you already have in your mind. You can start by asking questions like, "You said, you are an artist, what type of an artist are you?" "Where do you come from?" "What do you specialize in?" among others to help you gain some little confidence as well as experience slowly by slowly.

## Memorize a Few Questions

There are a set of questions that you can devote part of your free time to memorize. Such matters will play a very significant role when having a conversation with someone you are not familiar with. Additionally, those questions will instill some confidence in you given that you will always have something to fall back on during a conversation in any social setup. Having confidence is a critical factor that you will need to master if at all, you are looking forward to having your social skills top notch. This is the case, especially when you are faced with people that look intimidating to you. Portraying your social skills more confidently will set you way above everyone else in any social situation. It is good to understand the dynamics of a social world, and if you don't have the necessary skills, then you will not stand a chance to express yourself before other people.

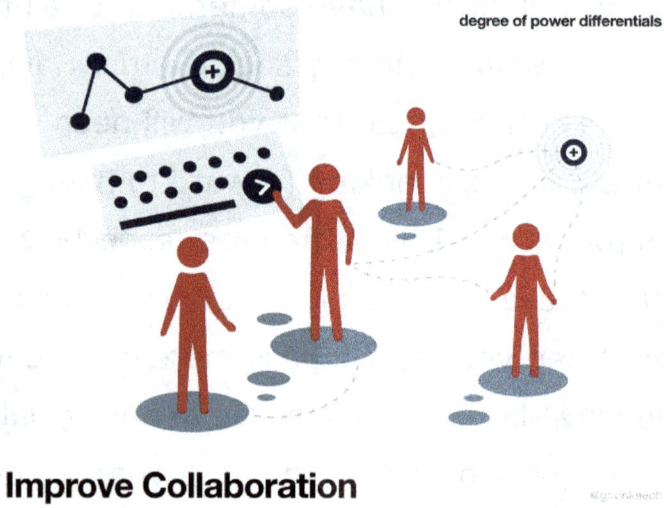
degree of power differentials
Improve Collaboration

## Learn a Few Tricks from Self-Confident People

Human beings are the smartest animals in the universe, but everyone learns new concepts, ideas, skills and actions from others. That is why there are role models, those who inspire and motivate others, and those who are celebrated because of what they have in their lives. That being said, there is no better way of learning a new idea or concept if not from someone you consider to be unique.

Take a good example of confident people in the showbiz and learn how they behave. Perhaps you are a great fan of James Bond, George Clooney, Oprah Winfrey or even Cristiano Ronaldo. It is no doubt that you consume a good percentage of your free time thinking, fantasizing, wishing and dreaming of being like one of these confident people. And the most exciting part of this observation is that you cannot afford to miss watching their films, their talk shows, listening to their interviews and reading about them in various magazines. What doesn't hit you is the fact that they are confident people and you can be like them if you learn how they carry themselves.

In reality, you should not think of faking who you indeed are unless you want to get a rude shock of your life shortly. Pretending self-confidence in a social situation may work for you at certain times but not always. Therefore, spend a little of your time and learn a few tricks from your role models, influential people and your peers. Make sure you apply what you have learned from others in a more appropriate way that will not bring you out as a fake person. No one likes associating with fakes. What it means by learning a few tricks from self-confident people is to get an overall idea of how you can confidently express yourself in a social situation. This can be done verbally, assuming a new posture, creating eye-contact, changing facial expression and using all necessary social values to gain an advantage over others.

Starting gradually to acquire social skills entails a lot, and you should be ready to venture further afield if you want to be seen as a social person. Even though you may face some difficulties along the way, it doesn't mean that you despair and fall out before achieving your goals. You should know that it takes a great sacrifice for one to succeed, and you should be ready to do what it takes for you to improve on your social skills.

CPSIA information can be obtained
at www.ICGtesting.com
Printed in the USA
LVHW081550250421
685458LV00009B/492

9 781801 679718